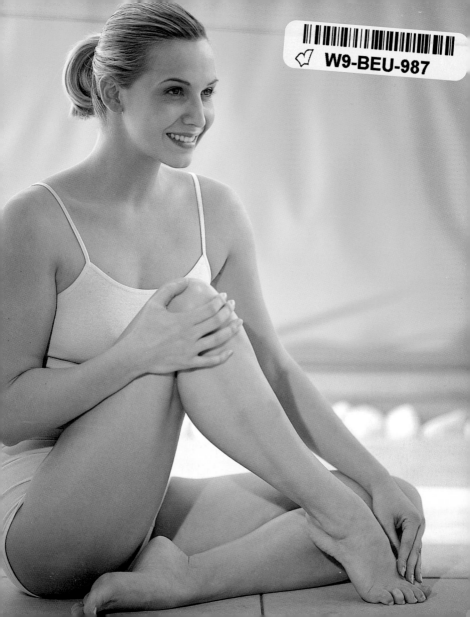

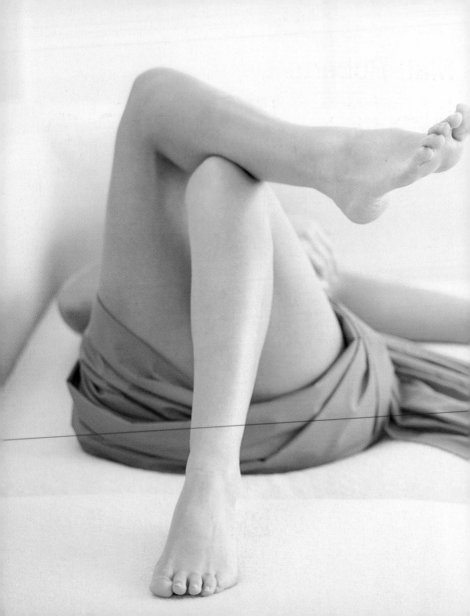

Matt Roberts
thin thighs

A DK Publishing Book

LONDON, NEW YORK, MUNICH,
MELBOURNE, and DELHI

This book is for my daughter Amber Lily

Editors Michael Fullalove, Anna Fischel
Project Art Editor Janis Utton
Managing Editor Gillian Roberts
US Editor Christine Heilman
Category Publisher Mary-Clare Jerram
Art Director Tracy Killick
DTP Designer Sonia Charbonnier
Production Controller Louise Daly
Photographer Russell Sadur

First American Edition, 2003
Published in the United States by
DK Publishing, Inc.
375 Hudson Street
New York, New York 10014

03 04 05 06 07 08 10 9 8 7 6 5 4 3 2 1

A Cataloging-in-Publication record for this book is available from the Library of
Congress.

ISBN 0-7894-9350-0

Color reproduced by GRB, Italy
Printed and bound in Italy by Printer Trento
See our complete product line at
www.dk.com

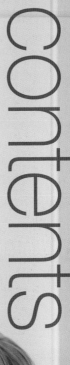
contents

about the book

It's one of those quirks of human biology that when a man puts on a few pounds, he gets love handles; and when a woman gains a bit of weight, she gets bigger hips and thighs.

It's not – naturally – quite so clear-cut as that, but it is true to say that a fair proportion of the women who come to see me have the same goal in mind – to lose their pear-shaped figures and to trim and tone their thighs. For all of them – and you – I've written this book, to share with you the secrets of getting leaner, longer-looking thighs.

I've created two special workouts. To do them, you don't need to set foot in a gym and you don't have to shell out for

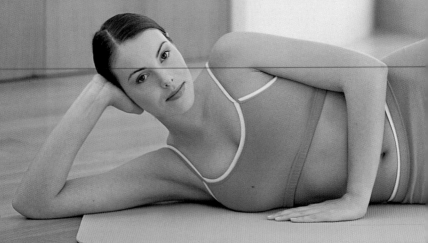

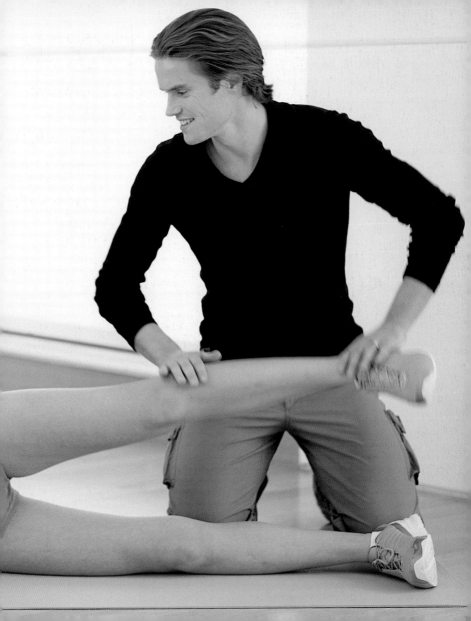

tons of fancy equipment. You can do them at home with the help of a jump rope, an exertube, and a fitness ball. (There's more on these last two on pages 92–93, along with some general information about using the workouts.)

To maximize their effect, the workouts themselves have a combination of approaches. There are dynamic moves like lunges and squats that work your lower body in its entirety. Other exercises target particular muscles (in your inner thigh, say). To burn fat and to sculpt your legs, there are short bursts of aerobic activity. I've also included some work for your buttocks (for a streamlined look) and a sequence of stretches that will keep your muscles looking long and lean.

And – because I know there's often more to getting gorgeous thighs than exercise alone – I'll be passing on the answers to those questions my clients ask me most, advising you on your technique, and giving you tips about healthy eating and such matters as the dreaded cellulite.

So, set aside 30 minutes every other day. Stick to my workouts. And fantastic thighs will be yours.
Here's to the new you,

Matt

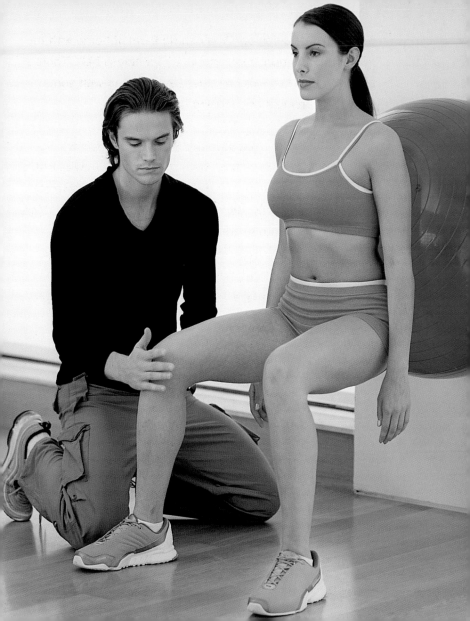

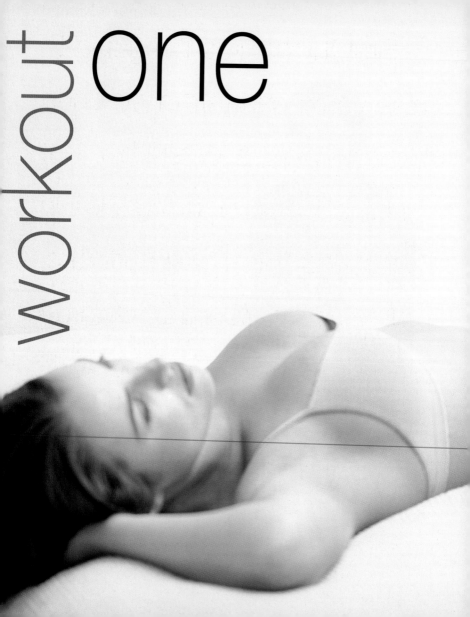

workout one

First things first: I'm going to raise your heart rate now. Then I'll keep it high, so you'll burn fat and condition the muscles in your legs, hips, and buttocks. Allow about 30 minutes to do this workout.

warm-up

Just before you start the exercises, you need to warm up for 5–10 minutes to prepare your body for the work ahead. Power walking or running are ideal choices because they burn fat and tone muscle. Do whichever feels most comfortable. Here are some tips for your technique.

• With power walking, make sure that when you're stepping forward, you plant your heel first, then roll through with your body weight. At the same time, bring your front hand up to about chest height (but don't lift it too high).

• When your weight is on your front foot, push your back leg into the stride (you should feel your buttocks and thighs working). Pull your other arm back strongly as you do so.

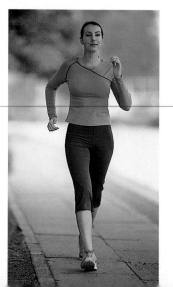

Running requires more power than walking. It's also high-impact, so wear good shoes. And make sure you:

• Take short, fast strides.

• Avoid high knee-lifts and big, bouncy steps (these will only tire you and strain your joints).

Once you've warmed up, move on to the basic squat.

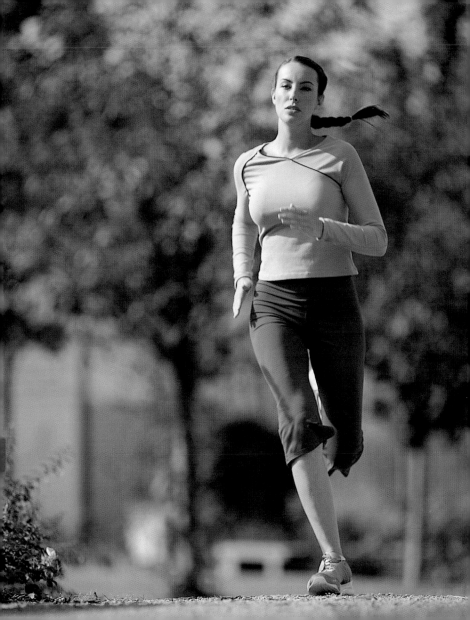

basic squat

A nice basic exercise that will raise your heart rate and get the major muscle groups of your lower body working hard.

level ①* do 10 squats
level ②* do 20 squats

1 Stand with feet hip-width apart and knees slightly bent. Keep your back straight and your arms relaxed by your sides.

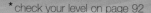

*check your level on page 92

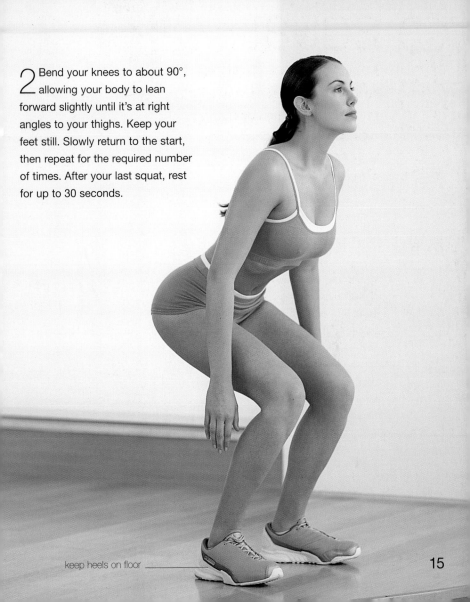

2 Bend your knees to about 90°, allowing your body to lean forward slightly until it's at right angles to your thighs. Keep your feet still. Slowly return to the start, then repeat for the required number of times. After your last squat, rest for up to 30 seconds.

keep heels on floor

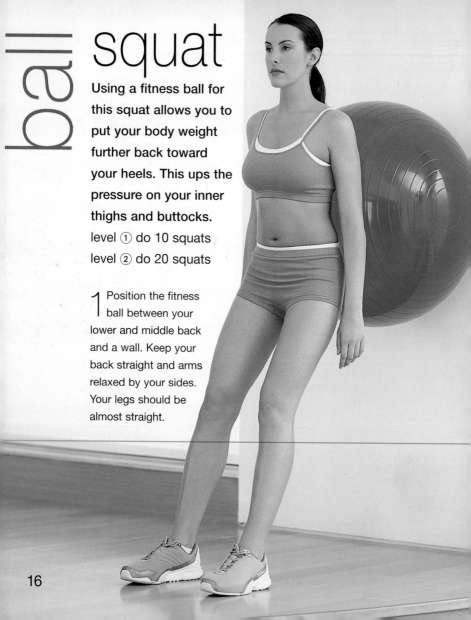

ball squat

Using a fitness ball for this squat allows you to put your body weight further back toward your heels. This ups the pressure on your inner thighs and buttocks.

level ① do 10 squats
level ② do 20 squats

1 Position the fitness ball between your lower and middle back and a wall. Keep your back straight and arms relaxed by your sides. Your legs should be almost straight.

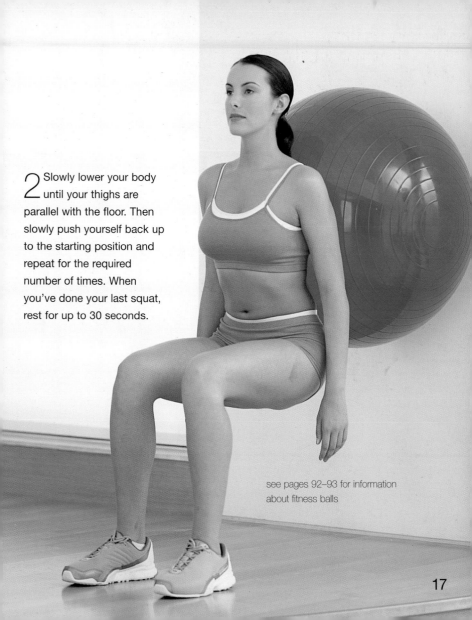

2 Slowly lower your body until your thighs are parallel with the floor. Then slowly push yourself back up to the starting position and repeat for the required number of times. When you've done your last squat, rest for up to 30 seconds.

see pages 92–93 for information about fitness balls

17

skipping

An old favorite of mine. Anyone can do this with a bit of practice. It's high-intensity and will definitely raise your pulse – a minute will be enough.

level ① do at least 50 skips

level ② do at least 70 skips

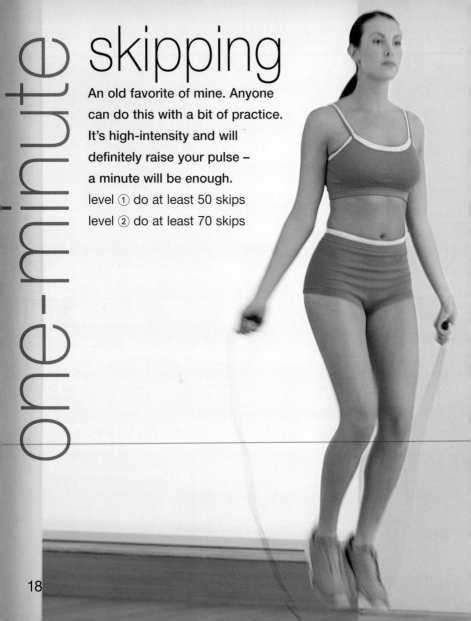

1 Stand with feet together and back straight. Hold the ends of the jump rope in your hands, with the rope behind your heels.

2 Pass the rope over your head and, as it approaches your feet, lightly bounce them off the floor. Try to keep both feet together and spring from the balls. Don't jump too high, though, since this can strain your knees. Continue until the minute is up, then rest for up to 30 seconds *(see right)*.

rests between exercises

Up till now I've told you when to take a rest between exercises. From now on, get into the habit of resting for up to a maximum of 30 seconds. Use these mini-breaks to take a sip of water – don't forget that your body dehydrates during exercise.

breathing correctly

One thing to keep an eye on is your breathing. Practice breathing in before you move and out as you move. Keep your tummy muscles taut and pulled in all the time. Above all, don't hold your breath! With continuous exercise such as skipping, try to breathe smoothly and rhythmically.

jump squat

The most advanced squat, to test your legs out completely. Let's see some air between your feet and the floor.

level ① do 10 squats

level ② do 15 squats

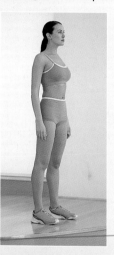

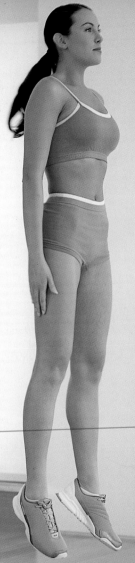

1 Stand with your feet hip-width apart, your back straight, and your arms relaxed by your sides. Bend your knees slightly, then jump up as high as possible.

2 Land on your toes, then lower your heels to the floor. Bend your knees and lower your body, imagining you're sitting down on a chair. Lean your body forward slightly, transferring your weight onto your toes. When your body is at right angles to your thighs, spring into the air again.

relax shoulders and keep them down

hands relaxed

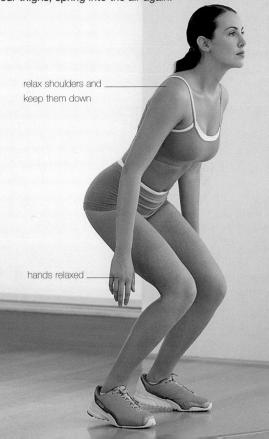

You're well into your stride now. Concentrate on getting your technique right – working your muscles in a thorough, effective way is far more important than hours spent overworking them. Thigh exercises are a relatively quick affair.

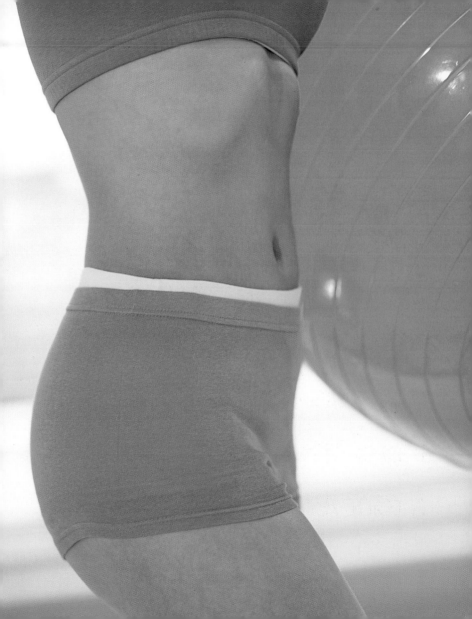

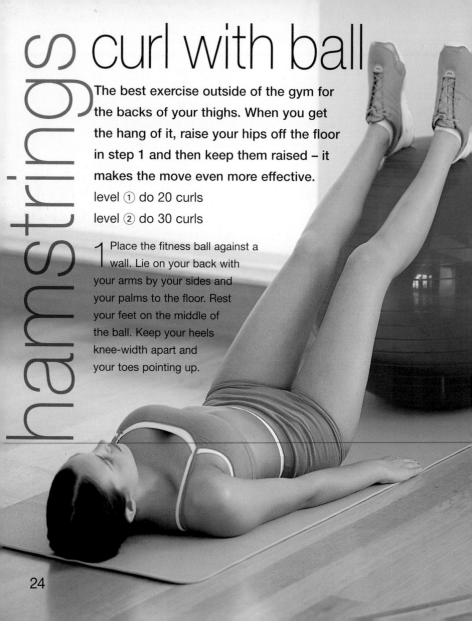

curl with ball

The best exercise outside of the gym for the backs of your thighs. When you get the hang of it, raise your hips off the floor in step 1 and then keep them raised – it makes the move even more effective.

level ① do 20 curls

level ② do 30 curls

1 Place the fitness ball against a wall. Lie on your back with your arms by your sides and your palms to the floor. Rest your feet on the middle of the ball. Keep your heels knee-width apart and your toes pointing up.

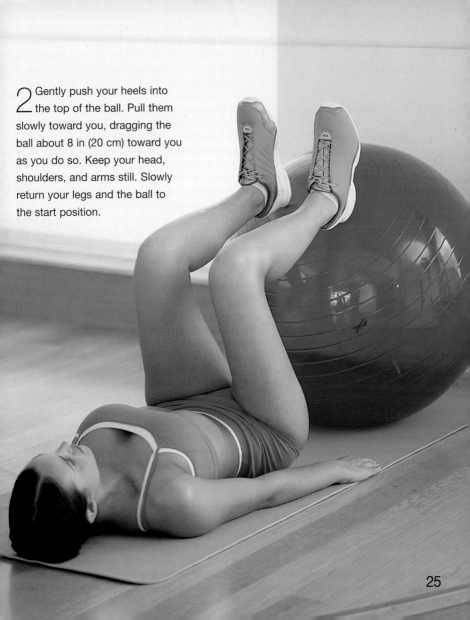

2 Gently push your heels into the top of the ball. Pull them slowly toward you, dragging the ball about 8 in (20 cm) toward you as you do so. Keep your head, shoulders, and arms still. Slowly return your legs and the ball to the start position.

25

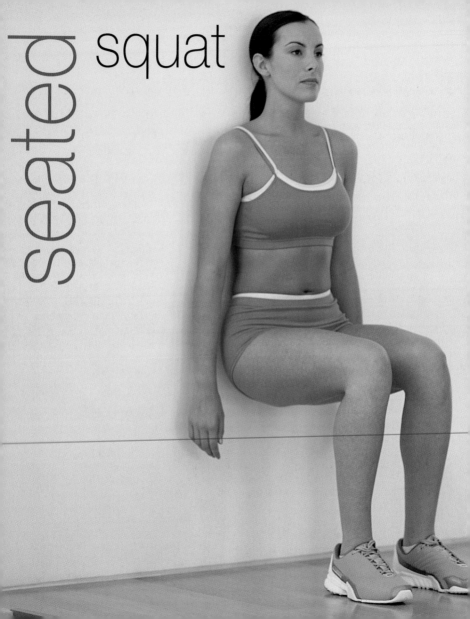

seated squat

An exercise skiers use. It may make your legs burn, but they'll be leaner, firmer, and stronger as a result.

level ① hold for 30 secs

level ② hold for 60 secs

Stand with your back flat against a wall and your feet about 12 in (30 cm) from it. Keep your arms relaxed by your sides. Slowly slide your body down the wall until your thighs are parallel with the floor. Adjust your foot position so your lower leg is completely upright, then pull your belly in toward your spine and hold the position still.

variation

avoiding the shakes

If you find this position too much of a strain and your legs start to wobble, walk around the room and shake your legs out before going on to the straight leg raise (page 30).

making it easier

The next time you do the seated squat, try lowering yourself down a little less, so your rear end stays higher up the wall and your thighs are at an angle. Hold the position for the correct length of time (or as long as feels comfortable). With practice, you should be able to lower yourself a little more each time. Eventually, you'll nail it.

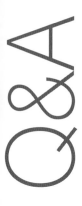

shaping up

How can I make my legs look longer?

Just keep on doing the lunges (like the forward lunge and the power lunge in workout two). These are great for making your legs look longer because they work the entire length of your thigh muscles rather than targeting just small areas of them. Concentrate on getting your technique just right. In addition, you could do some cycling. Or – if you belong to a gym – use the cross-trainer there. These activities will have the same effect.

My inner thighs are just about my worst feature. What can I do about them?

You'll be pleased to hear that you're already doing something about them. All the leg exercises in this book work your inner thighs. And better still, the inner thigh raise (pages 84–85) targets them specifically. Double the number you're doing if you'd really like to blitz them.

I have a pear-shaped figure and weight just pools around my hips and thighs. What can I do?

If your main concern is the weight you're carrying around your hips and thighs, I think you should focus on burning fat. Do this with some aerobic exercise. Then you can target the abductor muscles of your outer thighs and the glute muscles of your buttocks with raises that tone and firm them (*see pages 34–35 and 76–77*).

I haven't been able to wear my favorite pair of jeans for a couple of years now. How can I get back into them?

Whether it's your leg, hip, or waist measurement that's expanded, the best thing to do is combine the workouts in this book with a sensible eating plan and some extra aerobic exercise, such as cycling, swimming, running, or walking. Alternate this with the workouts, so your week might be: Monday – workout one; Tuesday – swim; Wednesday – workout two; Thursday – day off; Friday – workout one again; Saturday – 30-minute cycle ride; Sunday – workout two again. Also, make an effort to cut out unhealthy snacks and drinks and up your intake of water, fruit, and vegetables.

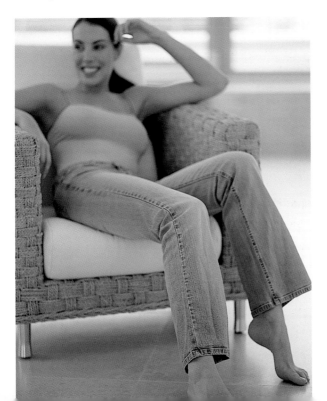

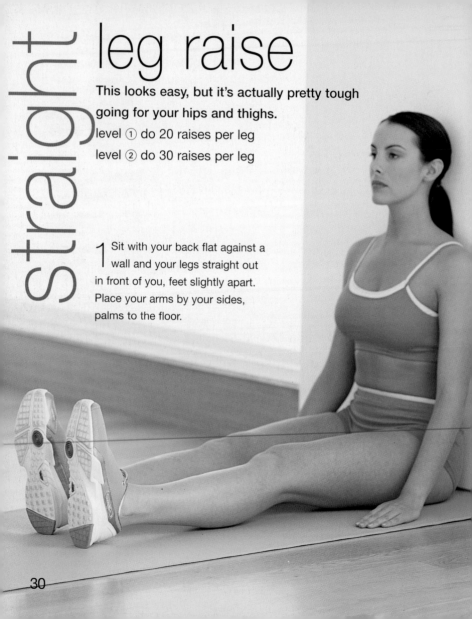

straight leg raise

This looks easy, but it's actually pretty tough going for your hips and thighs.

level ① do 20 raises per leg
level ② do 30 raises per leg

1 Sit with your back flat against a wall and your legs straight out in front of you, feet slightly apart. Place your arms by your sides, palms to the floor.

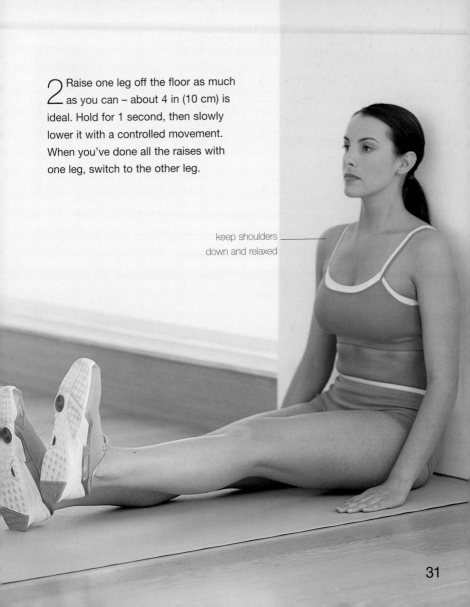

2 Raise one leg off the floor as much as you can – about 4 in (10 cm) is ideal. Hold for 1 second, then slowly lower it with a controlled movement. When you've done all the raises with one leg, switch to the other leg.

keep shoulders
down and relaxed

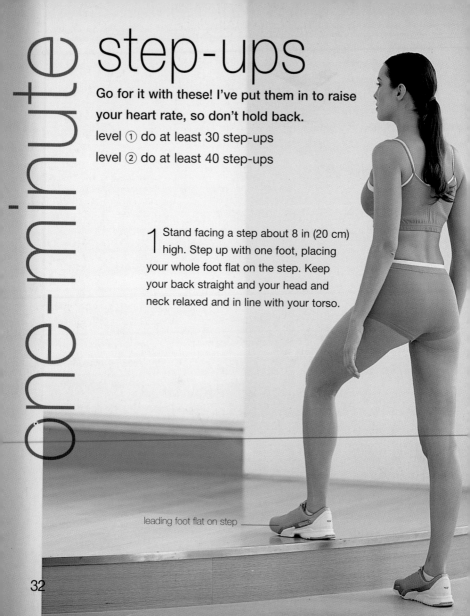

step-ups

**Go for it with these! I've put them in to raise
your heart rate, so don't hold back.**

level ① do at least 30 step-ups

level ② do at least 40 step-ups

1 Stand facing a step about 8 in (20 cm)
high. Step up with one foot, placing
your whole foot flat on the step. Keep
your back straight and your head and
neck relaxed and in line with your torso.

leading foot flat on step

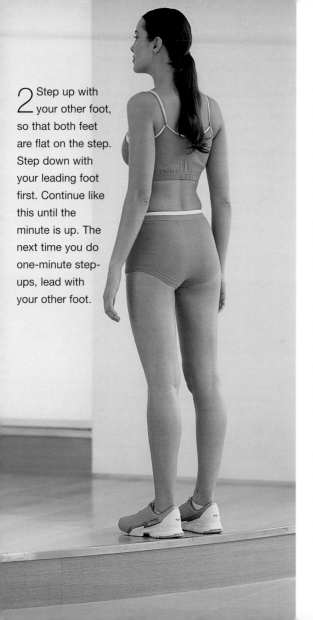

2 Step up with your other foot, so that both feet are flat on the step. Step down with your leading foot first. Continue like this until the minute is up. The next time you do one-minute step-ups, lead with your other foot.

eat lean

fat loss and calories

If you're trying to lose a few pounds while you trim and tone your thighs, keep a tight control over what you eat. Lower your daily intake by about 300–500 cal so your body's expending more energy than you're consuming.

exercise and calories

If you're not trying to lose weight, you should actually increase your calorie intake slightly when exercising. Eat an extra 300 cal each day.

a healthy diet

Whether you're counting calories or adding to them, you'll find a list of foods to eat more on page 67.

outer thigh raise

Try not to throw your leg around as you do this exercise.
Control the move with the muscles at the top of your hip and
in your buttock. Focus on these – you'll feel the work there.

level ① do 20 raises per leg

level ② do 30 raises per leg

1 Lie on one side with your upper
body supported on your forearm and
elbow. Place the other hand in front to
steady yourself.

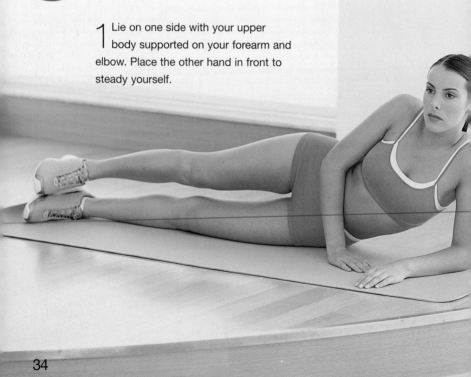

2 Keeping your leg straight and in line with your hip, raise it up with a slow and controlled movement. Hold for 1 second, then return to the start. Do all the raises with one leg, then turn over and do them with your other leg.

keep leg in line with body

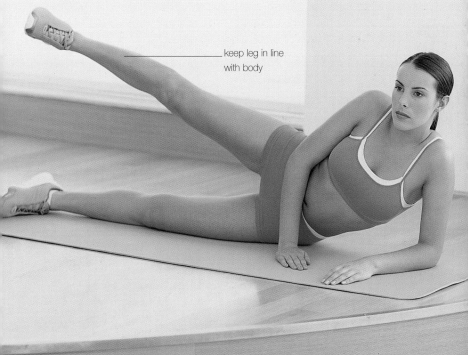

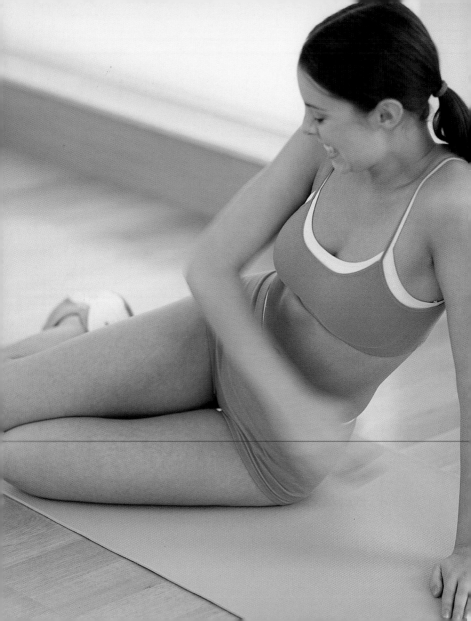

If your legs are starting to feel a bit tired and shaky, take a breather for a moment or two. If they're flagging but still working hard, you're right in the zone. Give yourself another little push – you may be surprised by how much energy you have in reserve.

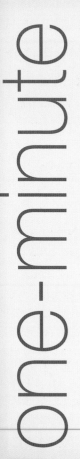

one-minute butt kicks

A quick exercise to get the hamstring muscles at the back of your thighs working. It's simple but very effective because of the number of kicks you're doing.

level ① do at least 50 kicks

level ② do at least 70 kicks

1 Stand with feet hip-width apart and hands at buttock-height behind you. Kick one leg behind you, aiming for your hands (you don't have to touch them).

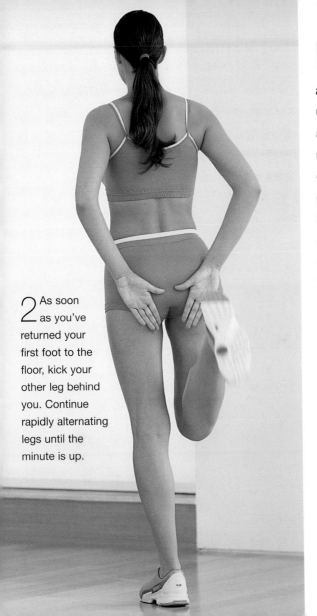

2 As soon as you've returned your first foot to the floor, kick your other leg behind you. Continue rapidly alternating legs until the minute is up.

body talk

about cellulite

Cellulite on thighs, buttocks, and arms is a concern for many women, whether they're overweight or not. Although genetics – and age – have a large part to play, there's much you can do to help eliminate cellulite, not least of which is exercise. There's even growing evidence that you can cut the risk of developing cellulite in the first place. For the answers to some of the most frequently asked questions, turn to pages 68–69.

exertube

leg extension

I've adapted this move from a classic gym exercise. If you're new to exertubes, you can read more about them on page 73.

level ① do 15 extensions per leg

level ② do 25 extensions per leg

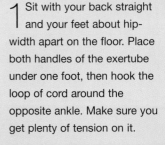

1 Sit with your back straight and your feet about hip-width apart on the floor. Place both handles of the exertube under one foot, then hook the loop of cord around the opposite ankle. Make sure you get plenty of tension on it.

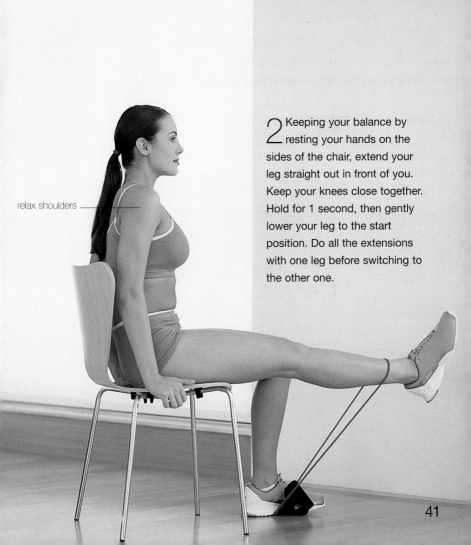

relax shoulders

2 Keeping your balance by resting your hands on the sides of the chair, extend your leg straight out in front of you. Keep your knees close together. Hold for 1 second, then gently lower your leg to the start position. Do all the extensions with one leg before switching to the other one.

41

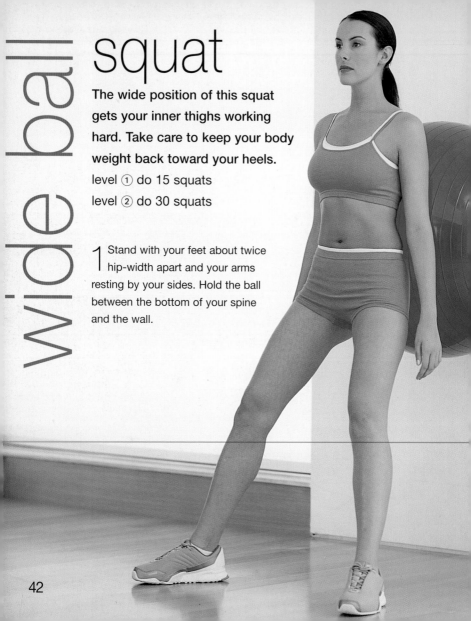

squat

The wide position of this squat gets your inner thighs working hard. Take care to keep your body weight back toward your heels.

level ① do 15 squats

level ② do 30 squats

1 Stand with your feet about twice hip-width apart and your arms resting by your sides. Hold the ball between the bottom of your spine and the wall.

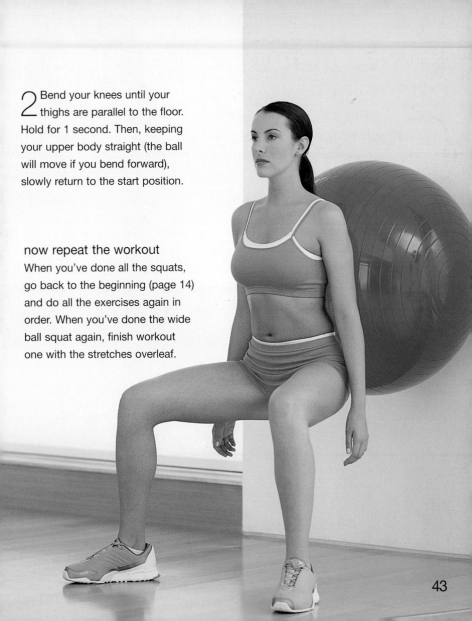

2 Bend your knees until your thighs are parallel to the floor. Hold for 1 second. Then, keeping your upper body straight (the ball will move if you bend forward), slowly return to the start position.

now repeat the workout

When you've done all the squats, go back to the beginning (page 14) and do all the exercises again in order. When you've done the wide ball squat again, finish workout one with the stretches overleaf.

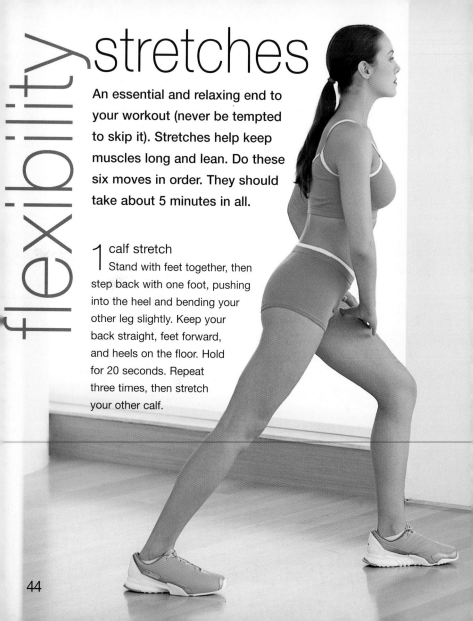

flexibility stretches

An essential and relaxing end to your workout (never be tempted to skip it). Stretches help keep muscles long and lean. Do these six moves in order. They should take about 5 minutes in all.

1 calf stretch
Stand with feet together, then step back with one foot, pushing into the heel and bending your other leg slightly. Keep your back straight, feet forward, and heels on the floor. Hold for 20 seconds. Repeat three times, then stretch your other calf.

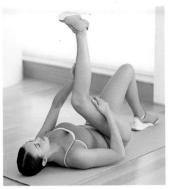

2 back of the thigh stretch

Lie on your back with your left leg bent and your foot flat on the floor. Hold your right leg with one hand behind the thigh and one behind the calf muscle. Keeping this leg as straight as possible, gently pull it toward you. Hold for 10 seconds, allowing the muscle to relax into the stretch. Repeat with the other leg.

3 buttock and thigh stretch

Lie on your back. Bend your right knee, keeping your foot on the floor, and cross your left leg over it, so your left ankle rests just above your right knee. Hold behind the right thigh with both hands and gently pull your leg toward you. Hold for 10 seconds, then repeat with your other leg.

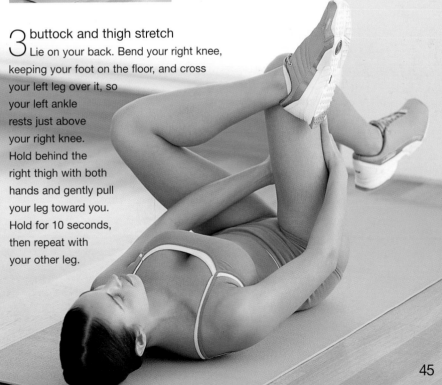

4 front of the thigh stretch

Lie face down. With hips on the floor, bring your right leg up behind you. Grip the foot and hold for 10 seconds. Repeat with your other leg.

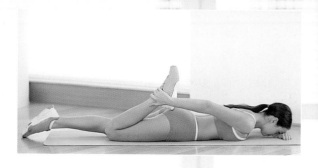

5 spine rotation

Lie on your back, with arms stretched out at shoulder level. Bend both legs to 90°, then drop your knees to the side so one knee is touching the floor. Keep your shoulder blades flat on the floor, but don't force the stretch. Hold for 15 seconds, then slowly return to the start position. Repeat on the other side.

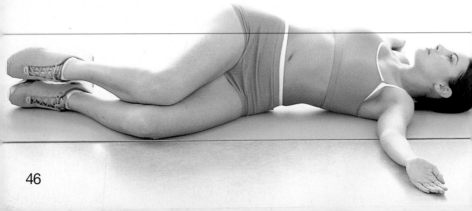

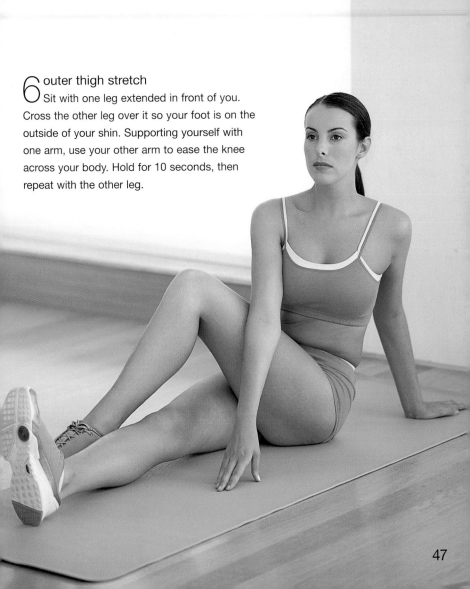

6 outer thigh stretch

Sit with one leg extended in front of you. Cross the other leg over it so your foot is on the outside of your shin. Supporting yourself with one arm, use your other arm to ease the knee across your body. Hold for 10 seconds, then repeat with the other leg.

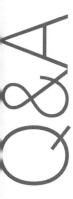

workout worries

I'm eager to work on my legs, but don't want to end up with big calf muscles. Am I in any danger of this with your workouts?

This is a question I'm always being asked, and quite rightly so. General leg workouts like mine tone your legs without making them bulky. That's because they combine dynamic exercises with short blasts of aerobic activity such as skipping to help the legs look longer and leaner. You're only at risk of developing big calf muscles if you continually target that area with one exercise – the step raise, say. So the answer is "no": these workouts of mine are designed to sculpt thin thighs not big calves.

I've just been sick in bed for a few days and couldn't face exercising. Will this be a setback?

This is nothing to worry about at all. There are times you shouldn't exercise, and when you're feeling exhausted and run-down is one of them. Your immune system has to work hard enough as it is when you're ill; don't deplete your body's reserves of energy further by exercising. Once you're up and around, try again with one of the workouts. But stop immediately if you start to feel dizzy or faint.

I like to alternate a home workout like these with a group activity. Which exercise classes are best for keeping my thighs toned?

Step classes are good for thighs, as is spinning (done on a stationary cycle). Most martial arts classes include a kicking element, which tones the legs. They're also great fun and really boost confidence. Try kickboxing, jujitsu, or capoeira, a dance-like Brazilian martial art performed to music.

Despite going on countless diets, my thighs stay as large as ever; it's my bust that gets smaller. What's going wrong?

The problem is "yo-yo" dieting: if you effectively starve yourself, your metabolism slows way down, so that any overeating when the diet is over really piles on the fat. It's better to develop a healthy eating plan that you can stick to. In your case, I suggest you exercise to shape up and speed your metabolism rather than reducing your calorie intake. Spend your nibbling time exercising and you'll kill two birds with one stone. You'll soon see results.

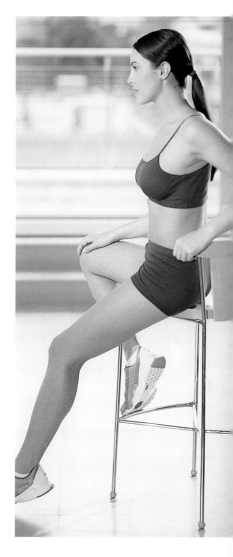

49

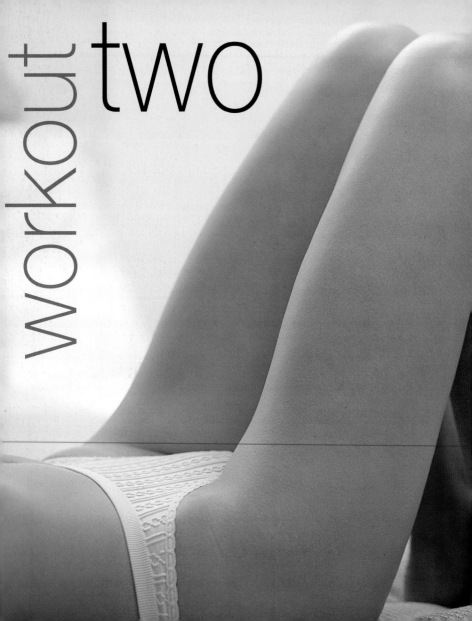

workout two

I'm stepping the work up a bit now – to tone your lower body more. Some of the exercises may feel quite intense, but stick with the program – the results will make it all worthwhile. Alternate this workout with the first one.

warm-up

To prime your muscles for the work to come, you need to warm up for 5–10 minutes, just as you did before workout one. If you chose to run at the last session, try power walking this time, and vice versa. Here are some more tips – they build on those I gave you on page 12.

When you're power walking, you're using your buttocks as workhorses to power you forward (which is why walking makes your bottom look lean and trim). Remember to:

- Keep your chin up and eyes ahead.
- Hold your tummy muscles tight.
- Keep your neck and shoulders relaxed.
- Avoid overstriding – keep your stride length short.

Running gets more enjoyable the more you do it. Make the most of it by paying careful attention to your technique.

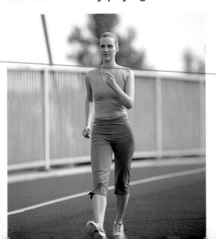

- Relax your shoulders.
- Use your arms to help your momentum. Swing them forward and backward (but don't exaggerate the motion).
- Keep your body upright and your tummy muscles pulled in tight.

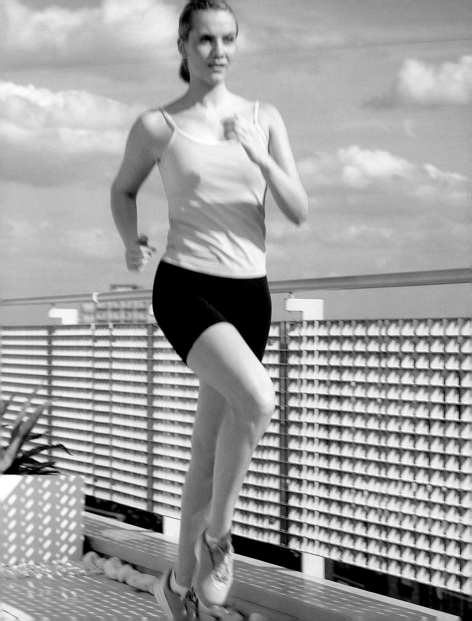

simple lunge

Another of my favorites. It's nice and simple, but it works your legs hard. Keep an eye on your posture.

level ① do 15 lunges per leg

level ② do 25 lunges per leg

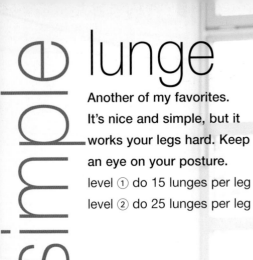

1 Place one foot in front of you about one stride-length from your back foot. Keep your hips facing straight ahead and your hands relaxed by your sides. Keep your body upright and your tummy pulled in.

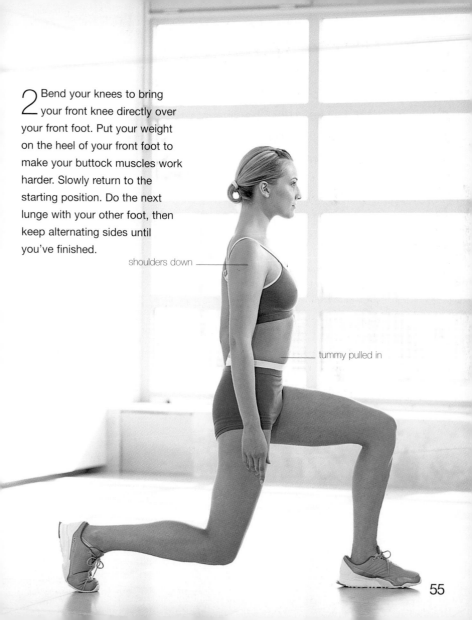

2 Bend your knees to bring your front knee directly over your front foot. Put your weight on the heel of your front foot to make your buttock muscles work harder. Slowly return to the starting position. Do the next lunge with your other foot, then keep alternating sides until you've finished.

shoulders down

tummy pulled in

55

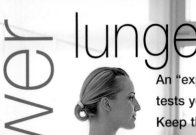

power lunge

An "explosive" version of the simple lunge that tests your legs and raises your heart rate. Keep the movement steady and controlled.

level ① do 15 lunges per leg
level ② do 25 lunges per leg

1 Stand with your feet hip-width apart and your hands relaxed by your sides. Keep your back straight, your tummy muscles pulled in, and your knees slightly bent.

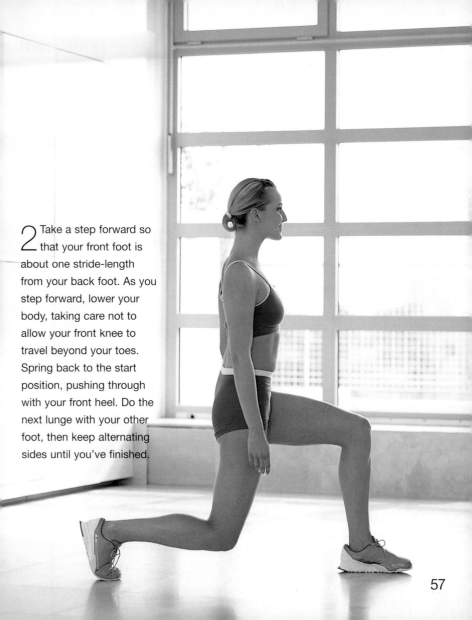

2 Take a step forward so that your front foot is about one stride-length from your back foot. As you step forward, lower your body, taking care not to allow your front knee to travel beyond your toes. Spring back to the start position, pushing through with your front heel. Do the next lunge with your other foot, then keep alternating sides until you've finished.

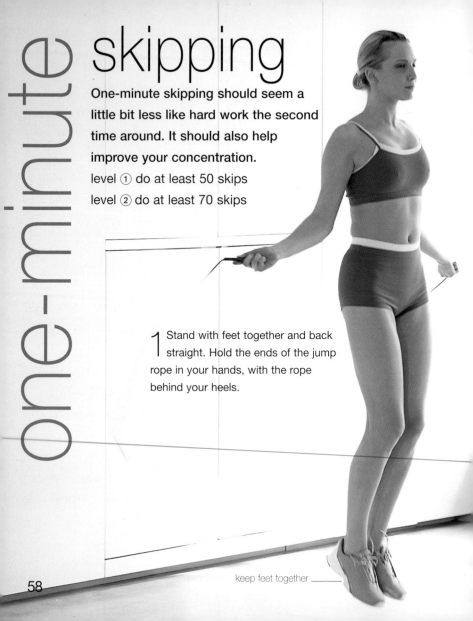

skipping

One-minute skipping should seem a little bit less like hard work the second time around. It should also help improve your concentration.

level ① do at least 50 skips
level ② do at least 70 skips

1 Stand with feet together and back straight. Hold the ends of the jump rope in your hands, with the rope behind your heels.

keep feet together

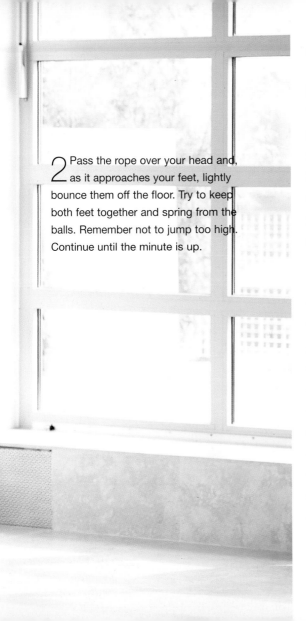

2 Pass the rope over your head and, as it approaches your feet, lightly bounce them off the floor. Try to keep both feet together and spring from the balls. Remember not to jump too high. Continue until the minute is up.

variation

tough on the knees?

The downside of jumping over the jump rope with feet together is that it can put strain on your knees. If your knees are your weak point and are beginning to feel a bit sore after one-minute skipping, try the boxers' "two-step" below.

the boxers' "two-step"

This lower-impact technique is used by boxers as part of their training. Instead of jumping over the rope with feet together, you transfer your bodyweight lightly from one foot to the other as you skip. Though it may take you some practice to perfect, your knees may well thank you for the effort.

When you're working your muscles hard, your body needs water, whether you're sweating or not. Get into the habit of taking a sip every few minutes, and be prepared to get through a pint or more during every workout.

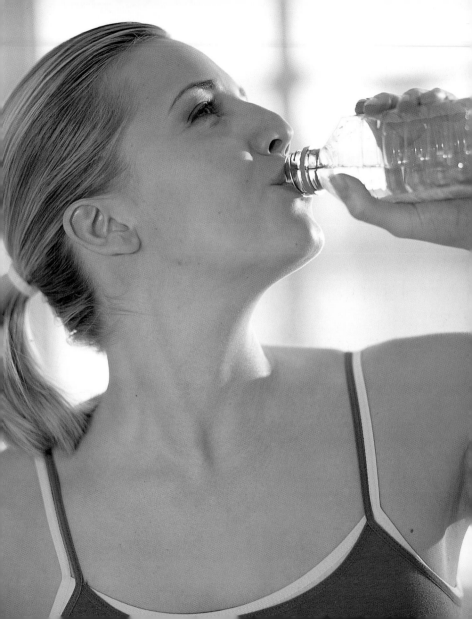

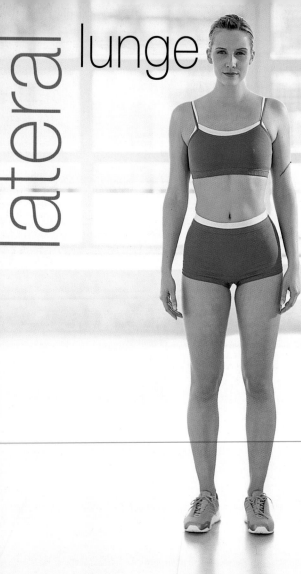

lateral lunge

This variation on the power lunge requires even more strength and control.

level ① 15 lunges per leg

level ② 25 lunges per leg

1 Stand with feet hip-width apart and back straight. Keep your hands relaxed by your sides.

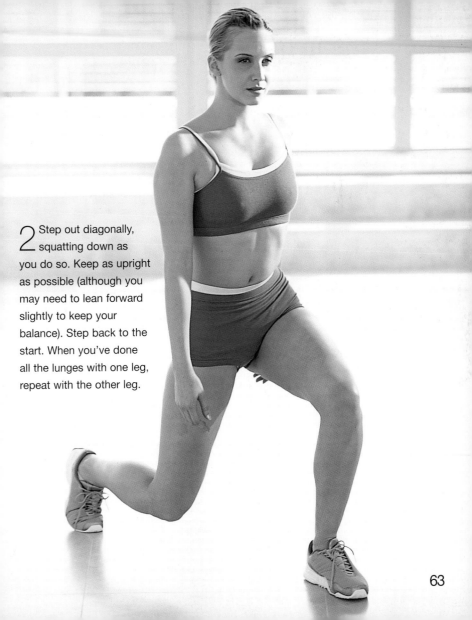

2 Step out diagonally, squatting down as you do so. Keep as upright as possible (although you may need to lean forward slightly to keep your balance). Step back to the start. When you've done all the lunges with one leg, repeat with the other leg.

forward lunge

You may need to clear yourself a bit of space for this exercise. Switch direction whenever you need to.

level ① do 20 lunges

level ② do 20 lunges

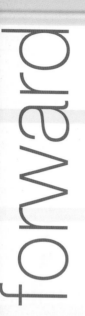

1 Stand with feet hip-width apart and knees slightly bent. Keep your back straight, your tummy muscles pulled in, and your hands relaxed by your sides. Step forward so that your front foot is about one stride-length from your back foot. Lower your body as you do this, then hold the position for 1 second.

knee no further forward than your toes

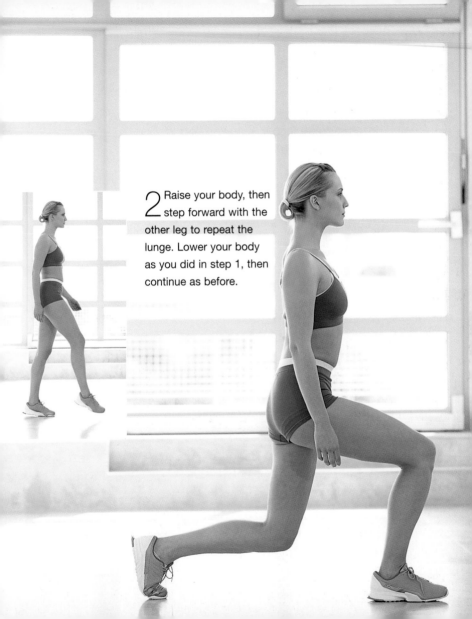

2 Raise your body, then step forward with the other leg to repeat the lunge. Lower your body as you did in step 1, then continue as before.

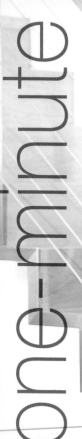

step-ups

Don't hold back again with the step-ups. You could even "jog" through them if you're feeling fit.

level ① do at least 30 step-ups

level ② do at least 40 step-ups

1 Stand facing a step. Step up with one foot, placing it flat on the step. Keep your back straight and your head and neck relaxed and in line with your torso.

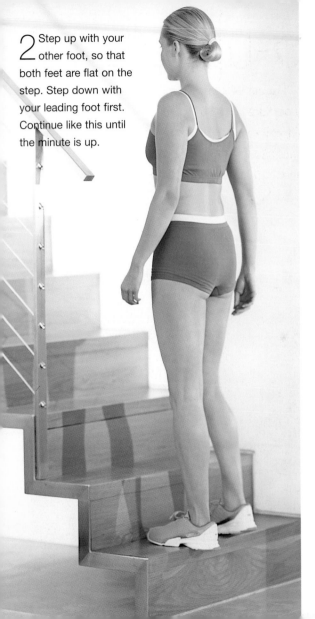

2 Step up with your other foot, so that both feet are flat on the step. Step down with your leading foot first. Continue like this until the minute is up.

eat lean

10 foods to eat more of

As much as I can, I try to eat foods that provide my body with slow-release energy. That way, I avoid the peaks and troughs that can lead to snacking. Alongside a plentiful supply of fresh fruit and vegetables, these 10 foods are my staples.

- brown rice
- whole-wheat pasta
- light rye bread
- dried beans and lentils
- chicken
- turkey
- firm white fish
- oily fish, such as salmon
- skim/soy/rice milk
- low-fat natural yogurt

(On page 83 there's a list of foods I avoid.)

banish cellulite

I'm getting cellulite on the backs of my thighs. Why is this happening?

Cellulite affects many people, men and women alike (although mainly women), and can develop on the buttocks and arms, as well as on the thighs. It's caused by toxins building up in fat cells. These then swell and push against the inflexible, meshlike connective tissue that holds the skin together. Cellulite's unmistakable dimpled "orange peel" appearance is the result. Don't despair about your cellulite, though – there are things you can do about it.

Does exercise help combat cellulite?

Regular exercise certainly helps, as does massage, which, by improving the circulation, helps rid the body of toxins. It also improves the elasticity of the connective tissue.

I've heard that a program of detox is good for cellulite. Is this true?

A detox program of a few weeks is an excellent way to cleanse fat cells. You can easily do it on your own. Start by drinking plenty of water. Then cut out – or at least reduce – coffee, tea, alcohol, and processed food. Replace them with fresh, preferably raw, fruit and vegetables and herb or fruit teas.

Ever since I lost puppy fat in my late teens, my legs have been thin but flabby. I do lots of walking, but that doesn't seem to make the saggy skin any tighter. What will help?

Skin naturally loses its elasticity the older you get. But exercise can help make it more springy, so keep going with the workouts. Also try massaging your legs, working upward from your feet and smoothing body lotion in as you go. In no time at all, you should feel relaxed in shorts and skimpy sportswear.

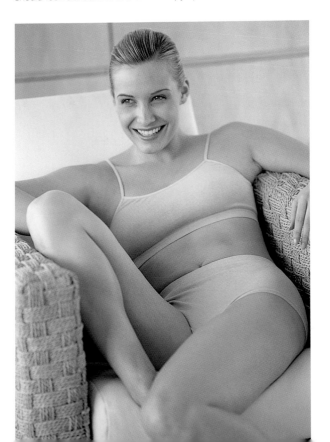

step raise

An exercise that targets your calf muscles. Don't worry that you'll end up making them beefy – the number of raises you're doing here will simply tone your legs.

level ① do 15 raises per side

level ② do 25 raises per side

1 Stand with the toes of one foot on a step. Hold on to something to keep your balance. Keep your back straight and your tummy in.

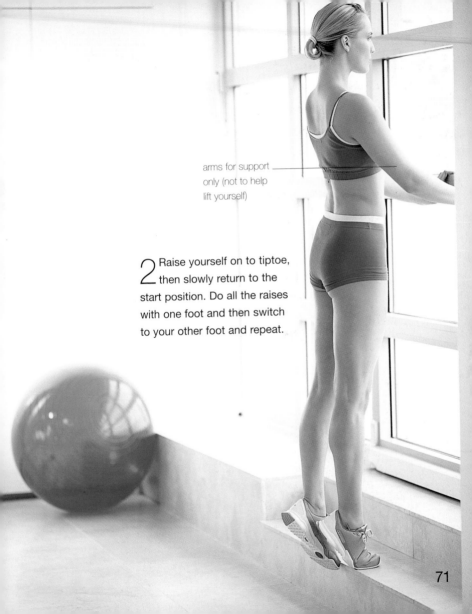

arms for support only (not to help lift yourself)

2 Raise yourself on to tiptoe, then slowly return to the start position. Do all the raises with one foot and then switch to your other foot and repeat.

hamstrings pull

Excellent work for the major muscle group at the back of your thigh.

level ① do 15 pulls per side

level ② do 25 pulls per side

1 Stand next to a wall or pillar. Secure both handles of the exertube under one foot, then hook the loop of cord around the heel of your working foot. Rest your hands on the wall and raise your foot off the floor slightly.

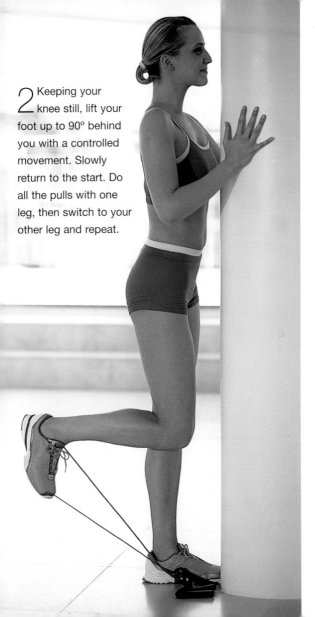

2 Keeping your knee still, lift your foot up to 90° behind you with a controlled movement. Slowly return to the start. Do all the pulls with one leg, then switch to your other leg and repeat.

about exertubes

This exercise is the second to use an exertube. I like them a lot because they're cheap, easy to use, and light.

which exertube to use

Exertubes come in color-coded strengths. Use a low-resistance tube if you're level ① and a medium-resistance one if you're level ②. Bear in mind that the exertube you use should allow you to perform the hamstrings pull and the exertube leg extension the correct number of times. It shouldn't be of such a low resistance that you're tempted to go on and perform more, or so high that you can't manage enough.

one-minute high knees

Performed quickly with good technique, this exercise tones your hip muscles to perfection.

level ① do at least 40 high knees

level ② do at least 60

1 Stand with feet hip-width apart and hold your hands out in front of you, elbows bent at right angles. Bring one knee up to hip-height, aiming to hit your hand with your knee.

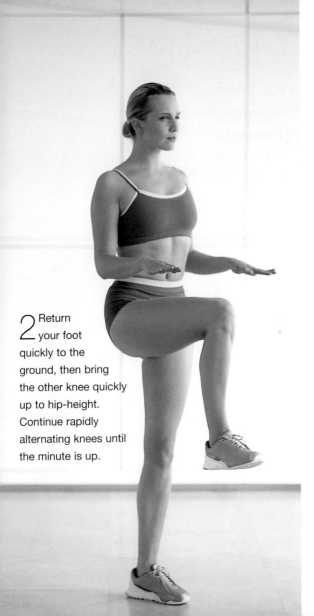

2 Return your foot quickly to the ground, then bring the other knee quickly up to hip-height. Continue rapidly alternating knees until the minute is up.

body talk

fears of bulking up?

Don't be alarmed if, 10 days into the workouts, your jeans feel a little tighter at the end of one of your sessions, or it feels as though your muscles are growing. They're not. At least, they may be, but it's just a temporary thing.

fluid retention

Sometimes when you're working your body hard, it holds on to fluids in your muscles to help them recover. This will pass, believe me. Your leg muscles will soon "dry out," leaving your thighs looking lean and feeling toned.

side raise

This might look a little strange, but it does work your hips and your buttocks intensively, provided you keep your body still and focus on squeezing your buttocks hard.

level ① do 15 raises per leg

level ② do 25 raises per leg

1 Get down on all fours, with your thighs at right angles to the floor and your knees hip-width apart. Keep your arms slightly bent and slightly wider than shoulder-width apart. Keep your head and neck in line with your spine.

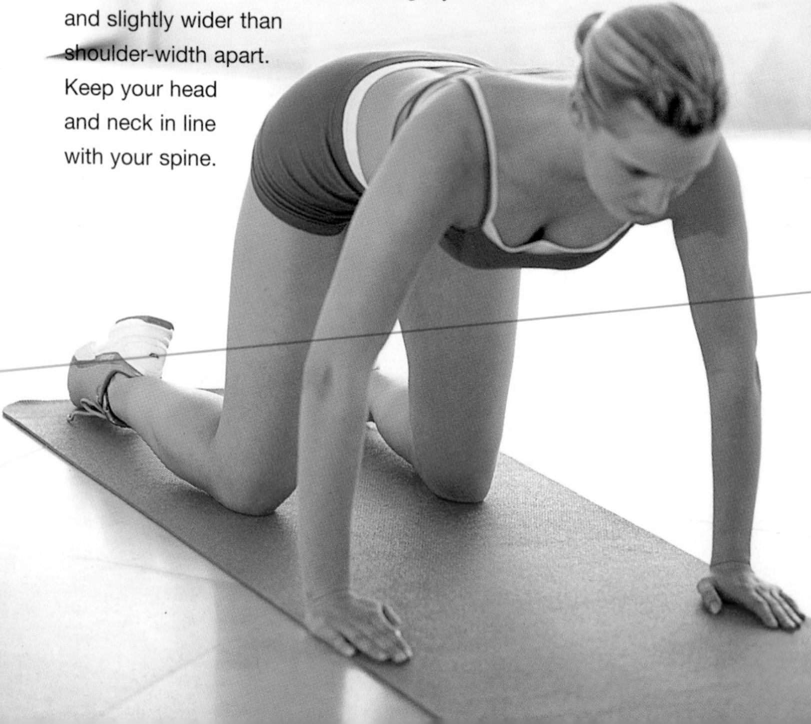

2 Squeeze your buttocks and move your knee out sideways. Lift it as far as you can without rotating your hips or twisting your back. Slowly return to the start. Do all the raises with one leg, then switch to the other leg and repeat.

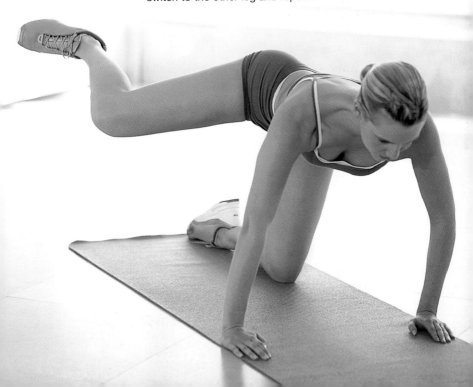

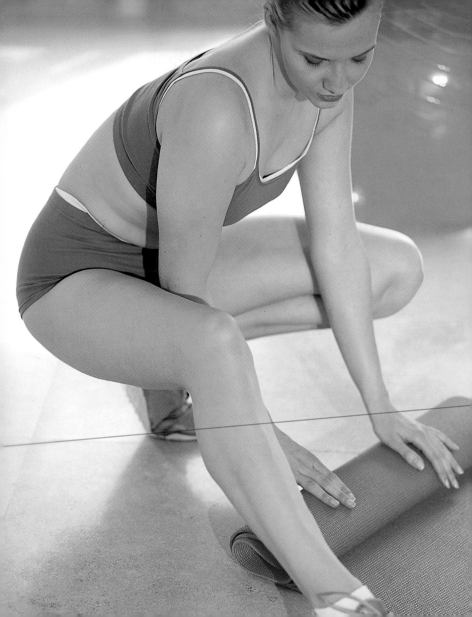

Do your best to think positive and stay motivated, even when the workouts seem tough. If you really want to make this work for you, give the extra 10%. Picture your legs in the shape you want them to be. Be realistic. And don't give in until you get there.

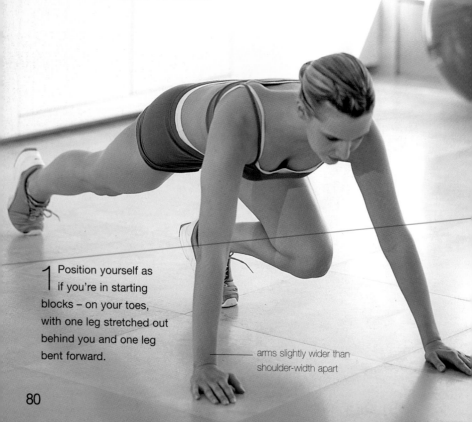

half squat thrust

Get the very most from this exercise by really driving your legs behind you. Keep your speed up, too, but not at the expense of your posture – your back should stay steady.

level ① do 20 thrusts

level ② do 40 thrusts

1 Position yourself as if you're in starting blocks – on your toes, with one leg stretched out behind you and one leg bent forward.

arms slightly wider than shoulder-width apart

2 Keeping your back as steady as you can, jump from one foot to the other, alternating which leg you're stretching out behind you and which leg you're bending forward. Stay on your toes and keep your neck relaxed and in line with your spine.

keep your
back steady

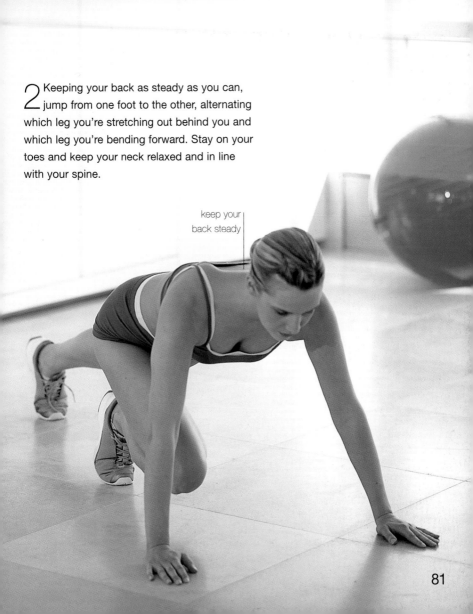

butt kicks

Time to give the hamstring muscles at the back of your thighs another blast.

level ① do at least 50 kicks

level ② do at least 70 kicks

1 Stand with your feet hip-width apart and hands at buttock-height behind you. Kick one leg behind you, aiming for your hands (but there's no need to touch them).

hips straight

2 As soon as you've returned your first foot to the floor, kick your other leg behind you. Continue rapidly alternating legs until the minute is up.

eat lean

10 foods to avoid

On page 67 I gave you a list of foods I eat all the time. Here's a list of those I avoid: they're sources of quick-release energy that rapidly fuel the body with 'sugar,' and just as quickly leave it wanting more. The danger then is snacking. Quite a few of the staples of western diets are on my list.

- bread made with wheat
- potatoes
- butter
- cheese
- whole milk
- alcohol
- chocolate
- tea & coffee
- chips
- processed food

thigh raise

You've been here before, I know: raising your legs every which way in a class. But this is a truly effective exercise and you'll love the results – great inner thighs.

level ① do 15 raises per side

level ② do 30 raises per side

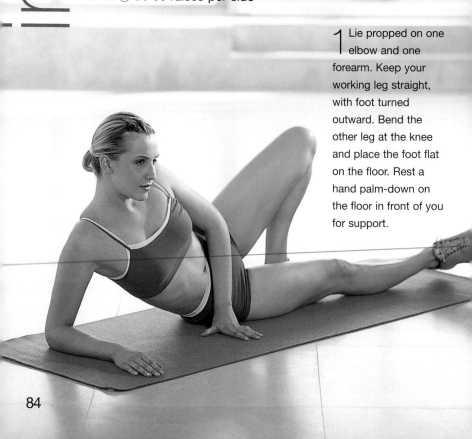

1 Lie propped on one elbow and one forearm. Keep your working leg straight, with foot turned outward. Bend the other leg at the knee and place the foot flat on the floor. Rest a hand palm-down on the floor in front of you for support.

2 Without moving your hips or your upper body, lift your working leg vertically as high as you can. Keep your foot flexed and your leg straight. Hold for a moment before slowly lowering your leg to the floor. Do all the raises with one leg, then switch legs and repeat.

now repeat the workout

When you've done all the raises, go back to the beginning (p. 54) and do all the exercises again in order. When you've done this raise again, finish workout two with the stretches overleaf.

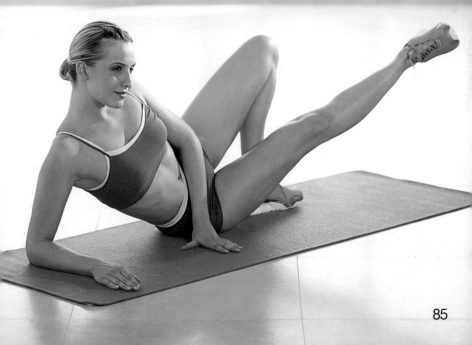

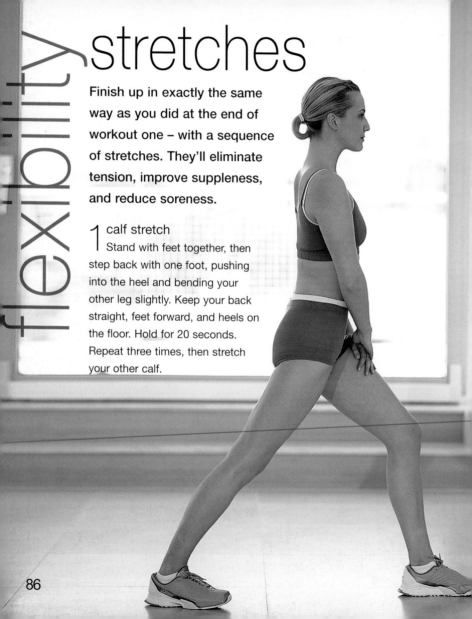

flexibility

stretches

Finish up in exactly the same way as you did at the end of workout one – with a sequence of stretches. They'll eliminate tension, improve suppleness, and reduce soreness.

1 calf stretch
Stand with feet together, then step back with one foot, pushing into the heel and bending your other leg slightly. Keep your back straight, feet forward, and heels on the floor. Hold for 20 seconds. Repeat three times, then stretch your other calf.

2 back of the thigh stretch

Lie on your back with your right leg bent and your foot flat on the floor. Hold your left leg with one hand behind the thigh and one behind the calf muscle. Keeping this leg straight, gently pull it toward you. Hold for 10 seconds. Repeat with your other leg.

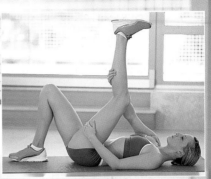

3 buttock and thigh stretch

Lie on your back. Bend your left knee, keeping your foot on the floor, and cross your right leg over it, so your right ankle rests just above your left knee. Hold behind the left thigh with both hands and gently pull your leg toward you. Hold for 10 seconds, then repeat with your other leg.

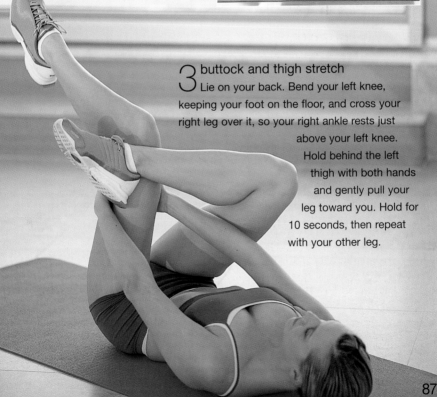

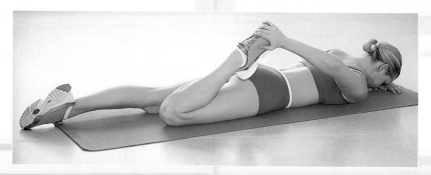

4 front of the thigh stretch
Lie face down with your hips on the floor. Bring your right leg up behind you, grip the foot, and hold for 10 seconds. Repeat with your other leg.

5 spine rotation
Lie on your back with your arms stretched out at shoulder level. Bend both legs to 90°, then drop your knees to the side so one knee is touching the floor. Keep your shoulders flat on the floor, but don't force the stretch. Hold for 15 seconds, then slowly return to the start. Repeat on the other side.

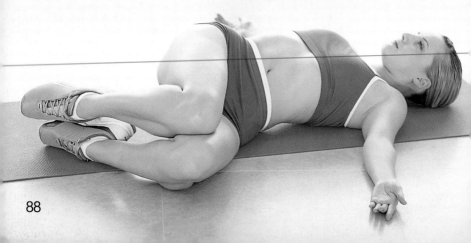

6 **inner thigh stretch**
Sit with your back straight. Place the soles of your feet together and, holding your ankles, pull your feet in toward you. Hold the stretch as your knees relax toward the floor. Intensify the stretch by placing your elbows on your knees and, keeping your back straight, gently easing your body forward from the hips. Hold for 10–12 seconds.

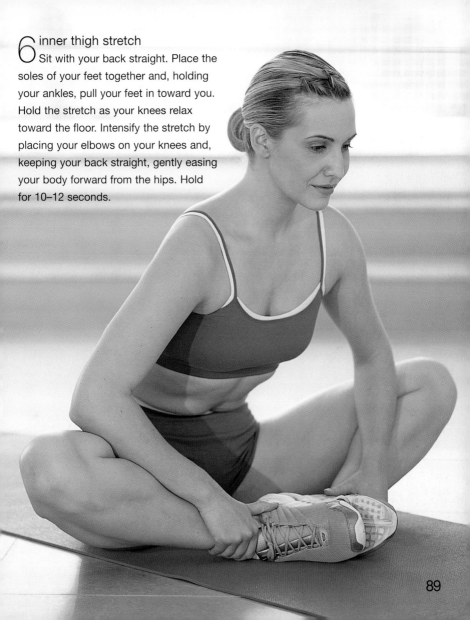

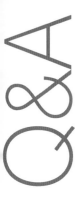

keeping it up

I'm finding it hard to keep my interest up. I've worked hard to get my thighs slim and really don't want to drift back to being the flabby old me. Do you have any suggestions?

You've done really well. Congratulations. And you're absolutely right to beware of complacency and boredom. These are two of the most common pitfalls. Luckily, keeping your thighs thin is a whole lot easier than getting your thighs thin in the first place. So cut yourself some slack: you're not going to have to exercise quite so often or quite so hard from now on. Keep your motivation high by varying your routine – instead of running and walking, try warming up by cycling or going for a swim.

When I started the workouts my legs ached afterward, but they don't at all now. Is this a good sign? Or should I be working harder?

It's both – you're getting fitter, but it's also time to move up a level. (This also applies if you've begun to find the workouts a bit on the easy side.) If you're currently on level ①, upgrade to level ②. If you're already on level ②, repeat the workouts twice rather than just once. And make sure you're doing the exercises correctly – sloppy work makes for a sloppy body.

My friend suggests we start exercising together, but I'm worried we won't take it seriously. What do you think of the idea?

Anything – or anyone – that encourages you to exercise (including a talkative training buddy) is a good idea in my book. You've got someone to keep you motivated and someone to ensure that you train when you say you're going to. I suggest you keep the pace up so neither of you has the breath for too much chatting!

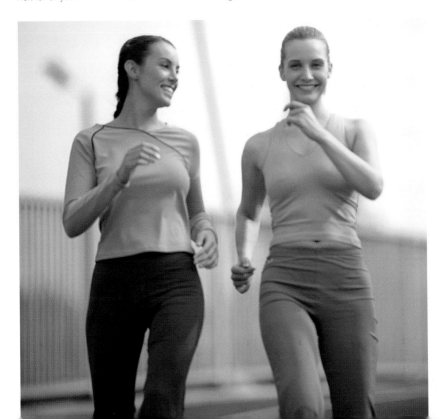

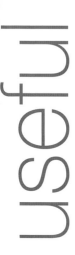

information

which fitness level?

Before you start the workouts, you need to know your fitness level – ① or ②. If you're currently getting little or no exercise, start at level ①. If you already do 30 minutes or more aerobic exercise (that's enough to make you puff and sweat) three times a week, start at level ②. If you're a level ① user and you start to find the routines too easy, upgrade yourself to level ②. Similarly, level ② users who start to find the routines a cinch should repeat each workout twice all the way through rather than just once.

how often to peform the workouts

Aim to perform each workout twice a week. Do them alternately.

the equipment you need

Apart from a jump rope and an exercise mat (you might not even need that if you're working on a carpet) there are just two pieces of equipment you need – a fitness ball and an exertube.

fitness balls You'll sometimes see these called Swiss balls, stability balls, gym balls, back balls, or birth balls. I think they're great: they make exercise fun and improve your balance as well as toning your muscles. They come in three sizes according to your height and weight. The medium size is correct for most women (though you may prefer to get the small size if you're under 5 ft 2 in/1.55 m). You can buy them from most sports shops and department stores, but in case you have any problems tracking them down, I've given you some suppliers below.

exertubes These have other names too, like resistance tube, exercise band, and fit-tube. They're an extremely versatile piece of equipment, but for the workouts in this book I've given you pretty much all you need to know on page 73. They're generally available from most of the same outlets that sell fitness balls, but for other suppliers see below.

suppliers of fitness balls and exertubes

If you have problems finding fitness balls and exertubes in your local stores, you can order them from:

In the US
Ball Dynamics
800 752 2255
www.balldynamics.com

In Canada
IncrediBall Enterprises Ltd
Toll free 1 877-348-2255
www.incrediball.ca

index

author's credits

Thanks to everybody (too many of you to name, alas) who helped me with this book. A special thank you to the DK team, to Michael, Tracy, and Anna, in particular; to Russell for the great shots; to my own team, especially Nik, Richard, Jason, Ayo, and Alan; and to my brother Jon, who, as always, shared the workload with me. For more information about Matt Roberts Personal Training, please contact:

matt roberts personal training

32–34 Jermyn St

London SW1Y 6HS, UK

Tel: 011-44-207-439-8800

www.personaltrainer.uk.com

publisher's credits

Thanks to our models Janine Newberry and Kirsty Spence from ModelPlan, and to Nessie at ModelPlan; to Matt's team of trainers: Nik Cook, George Dick, Jason Hughes, Ayo Williams, and Alan Foley; to Toko at Hers and to Cor Kwakernaak for hair and makeup; to stylist Jo Atkins-Hughes; and to photography assistant Nina Duncan. Many thanks to Reebok (1-866-271-5859) for the kind loan of shoes for this book and to Agoy (011-44-208-933-8421 or www.agoy.com) for the kind loan of the exercise mats.

about the author

Matt Roberts, the UK's hottest personal trainer, began as an international sprinter. He went on to complete his studies at the American Council for Exercise and the American College of Sports Medicine. Affectionately known as "the personal trainer to the stars," Matt has an enviable reputation for training celebrities, among them Sandra Bullock, Trudie Styler, Mel C, Natalie Imbruglia, Naomi Campbell, Tom Ford, John Galliano, and Faye Dunaway. Alongside this high-profile client list, Matt derives equal satisfaction from helping each of his clients meet their health and fitness goals. And in his quest to make fitness and good health accessible to everyone, he produces his own range of vitamins, home gym equipment, and body care products.